99 Natural Ways to Beat a Headache

Your Headache Pain Can Be Stopped, With Simple But Very Effective Strategies And Without Resorting To Drugs.

DISCLAIMER AND/OR LEGAL NOTICES:
The information presented herein represents the view of the author as of the date of publication. The report is for informational purposes only.
While every attempt has been made to verify the information provided in this report, neither the author nor his affiliates/partners assume any responsibility for errors, inaccuracies or omissions or for any damages related to use or misuse of the information provided in the report. Any slights of people or organizations are unintentional. If advice concerning medical or related matters is needed, the services of a fully qualified professional should be sought. Any reference to any person or business whether living or dead is purely coincidental.

The Reason For This Book:

My name is Dr. Kelly Dullenty and I am a practicing Doctor of Chiropractic in the Southern United States. Since I started practicing, I have seen thousands of patients and have battled with countless conditions that keep people from having a normal life.

Some of the most common complaints I have come across in my time in practice, relate to the various types of headaches. This should come as no surprise being that nearly everyone has experienced a headache at some point in their life.

The reason this book exist, is that over the years I have discovered that, while some types of headaches are serious and require serious medical attention, the vast majority are simply caused by bad habits.

These bad habits are typically something that a person is doing on a daily basis and has done over and over for years. The problem with these bad habits is that the majority of the time, they end up causing major issues. This book is designed to help you, the reader, to eliminate those bad habits and, in turn, eliminate the core cause of your headaches.

This book is not meant to be a promotion for Chiropractic or Traditional medical treatments. This book is designed to help you eliminate the causes of your headaches so that you don't end up having to go to a doctor in the first place. Let's get started with a little background information on headaches.

FACT: Headaches Affect Nearly 90% of Men and 95% of Women

All kinds of pain are bad, but there is nothing as mentally exhausting as a headache. It affects our well-being, our productivity and even our social existence. After a headache, we feel mentally drained and physically exhausted. These annoying, painful, and sometimes intense episodes bring us to an interesting question: **Should a bad headache keep a good man (*or woman*) down?** To find a solution to this question, it is important that we understand more about headaches.

The most common types of Headaches can be identified as migraine, sinus, and tension. Now these headaches are very different, but they do affect the same part of the body--that is, the head in general. So if we understand more about them we can reach an interesting conclusion… Do you know what that is? Headaches are largely ***preventable***. Of course, there are a lot of cures available over the counter now, but do we really have to wait for the headache to start to resort to treatment? Isn't prevention better than cure? Isn't it better to be ***proactive*** than reactive?

I have included 99 tips on how to prevent headaches below. But before we go to the tips, it might be useful to have at least a superficial understanding of the different types of headaches.

Migraine Headaches

A migraine is a splitting headache that just seems to set in apparently due to no reason at all. The reasons for a migraine are mainly vascular. That means that certain changes in the blood vessels that supply blood to the brain trigger of the pain. Of course, the causes for the changes in the blood vessels may vary from person to person, but this is generally how it starts.

Migraines are easily the most common headache syndrome. They affect 10 to 15 percent of the global population. One peculiar feature of migraines is that they usually start in childhood or adolescence and are most common in young and middle-aged adults. Fortunately, one of the "perks" we are given for aging is that migraines usually stop as people get older.

These headaches have a strong impact on the quality of a person's life. They not only affect the person, but also the lives of those who live and work in close contact with that person. Migraine attacks can sometimes be so severe that person may have to abandon his or her routine activities for three or four days at a time. This can have a direct impact on family and co-workers of the migraine sufferer.

Once the pain of a migraine sets in, it is sheer agony. It is almost as if one side of your head is being ripped off and there is very little a person can do to stop this pain. If there is anything you can call "good" about a migraine, it is that they are transient, meaning the pain will go away after sometime. This usually happens after the person gets a few hours of sound sleep. However, one of the worst things about migraines is that they recur. Fortunately, migraines can be prevented to a very large extent as the following tips will explain.

There are two main types of migraine, the classic migraine and the common migraine. With the *classic* migraine an *aura* is present. This aura is the symptoms and feelings you have prior to the onset of the migraine. These aura symptoms may include blindness in half of your visual fields in one or both eyes, seeing flashes of light, blind spots, weakness, and skin paresthesia. Classic migraines make up about 20% of the migraine headaches that occur. The *common* migraine has some of the same symptoms as the classic migraine, but with out the aura. Common migraines make up the other 80% of occurring migraine headaches. Both the classic and the common kind can occur as often as several times a week or as rarely as once every few years.

Both types can happen at any time, but for some people, it *is* possible to predict when the occurrence of a migraine is going to happen. For example, certain migraine sufferers may know that they have a greater tendency for a migraine near the days of menstruation or maybe every Saturday morning after a stressful week of work.

Although many sufferers have a family history of migraine, the exact hereditary nature of this condition is not known. People who get migraines are thought to have an inherited abnormality in the regulation of blood vessels. The following factors often act as triggers that set of the migraine:

- **Stress**. This is one of the major factors that can contribute to the onset of a migraine. Knowing this is helpful, but it may not be possible for you to get away from the cause of stress, particularly if it is something connected with your job.

- **Anger**. This can be a huge trigger of a migraine as well. It is always a plus for short-tempered people to learn ways of controlling their anger. The best method is of course the 1 to 10 method. The next time you feel anger coming on, count to ten very slowly before you really blow your lid. By the time you get to ten you should have cooled down.

- **Physical and mental fatigue**. Both can lead to a migraine, so do not push your self too much. *Enough is enough*. When your body starts giving you signals that it has had enough, take heed and stop whatever you are doing. Just bear in mind that a little less productivity on one day is not worth the productivity of the next couple of days.

Sinus Headaches

Sinus problems give rise to a particular type of headache. The sinuses are small spaces in the facial bones just below the facial skin. The spaces are concentrated in the nasal region, temples and around the eyes. We have sinuses for a number of reasons: to reduce the weight of the skull, aid in smelling and breathing, protect the brain from blows to the face, and to aid in speech. Sometimes, due to infection, these spaces get inflamed with mucus and in turn, get infected as well.

This infection, known as *sinusitis,* often leads to a headache that feels like pressure. There are many causes for sinusitis which are allergy, a deviated nasal septum, severe cold, enlarged parts inside the nose, and acute ongoing infection.

Tension Headaches

Tension headaches are also common in many people. Stress and anxiety are major causes for these types of headaches. The moment a tension headache sufferer gets worked up about something, the person develops a tension headache. Lots of times this tension begins with a tightening of muscles in the neck and works its way into the head. Insufficient sleep, anxiety, problems, and worries give rise to this type of headache.

99 Tips

Now whatever the cause, or whatever the nature of the headache, most headaches are preventable. There is no need to endure the pain when you really have an option. Follow the tips given below and you will be amazed to find that the prevention *is* actually in your hands.

Tip 1.

Do not read when you are laying down. Try to avoid this at all cost. This posture is clearly *not* the best position for reading. It forces your neck into an undesirable position and likely will cause muscle tension and nerve pressure as well vascular compression. Flopping down on the bed with a book to read is very common. In fact, many people make it a habit to read for a few minutes before going to sleep. However, being in this position is a likely precursor for a headache to develop so let's just say it once and for all: It is *not* good to read while you are in the laying down position.

Tip 2.

Use pillows. Alright, I get it. For some of you this is the only way you can wind down after a stressful day and you are not going to give up reading while you lay down. So if you *must* read while lying, prop up your head with at least two pillows. Pillows give support to your head and neck so that your head is in a partially raised position. This will cause less harm to your eyes, neck and your head in general.

Tip 3:

Use adequate lighting. It is very important that you have a well-light room to read, do needle work, or any other such fine activity. Having the appropriate amount of light will limit the amount of stress put on your ocular and neck muscles. It should be noted that *too much* light is just as bad as a dimly lit room.

Tip 4.

Position the lighting appropriately. The source of light should preferably be behind your head when reading or doing work on a computer, and should not come in front of your eyes. The source of light should always be from behind you. Appropriate position of lighting will also inhibit eye strain and muscle strain of the neck.

Tip 5.

Do not hold objects too close. It is very natural for a person to bring a book or work they are doing close to their eyes in order to see print or detail better. This is bad for your eyes. Your eye muscles have to strain a lot in order to focus on nearer objects. The object should ideally be at the level of your chest.

Tip 6.

Do not hold objects too far away either. Holding things too far away is as bad as holding them too close. Remember, to keep it at chest level. Many bookstores have reading stands that will enable you to keep your book position at the right level. Positioning of the book or work you are doing is *very* important in prevention of headache pain.

Tip 7.

Pay attention to your eyes. If you find it difficult to read, get your eyes tested by an *eye specialist*. If you find yourself squinting or your eyes watering while you read or do any fine work, then you might need glasses. Do *not* waste time. Consult a doctor at the earliest time possible. Faulty vision is a *major* cause of headaches.

Tip 8.

Read with adequate print. Do not compromise your eyes if the print of the book is too faint or if the font size is too small. Most libraries and book stores have large-print versions of books. If this is not available, use a magnifying glass or wear magnifying glasses.

Tip 9 .

Do not read in moving vehicles. Many people try to read while traveling by car to pass time. However, curves and bumps in the road can cause headaches and even motion sickness. No matter how smooth the road and how good the shock absorbers of the car are, there is bound to be jerking motions. This will force your eyes to adjust and readjust to the print and this continuous adjustment and readjustment is very bad for your eyes. At the end of the journey you are bound to end up with a headache.

Tip 10.

Do not read from light of your TV or the monitor of your computer. This is not sufficient light to read, and your eyes will not be able to pick out what is printed. You should always use a lamplight or overhead light if you are reading while the TV is on or using your computer.

Tip 11.

Give your eyes a break. Your eyes will give you signs when they are under strain. You will find that you are getting tired sooner, your eyes may start to water or you might notice that you have to squint in order to get a better view. While doing work that requires you to strain your eyes, take breaks every *five* minutes. This is especially true for jobs like needle work and works involving electronic gadgets. This will give your eye muscles time to rest and regroup as well as help with neck tension from eye strain. The best relaxation for your eyes is staring at a distant object or just keeping them closed.

Tip 12.

Use an anti-glare screen. Anti-glare screens cut down the radiation you are exposed to from working on your computer. Radiation causes a great deal of harm to your eyes and an anti-glare screen is the best solution for this issue. If you are unable to use a screen, another option is to wear glasses that have an anti-glare coating on the lenses. It is also relevant that the glare from a computer alone can be huge triggers for headaches.

Tip 13.

Use lamps. If your job requires long hours in front of the computer, you may want to consider buying a special lamp that clips on the monitor. This lamp reduces the eye-strain caused by staring at the computer screen, and thus reduces headaches.

Tip 14 .

Eat plenty of carrots (or other foods high in beta carotene like sweet potatoes, mango, pumpkins, apricots and cantaloupe). They are especially good for your and are the best things that nature has to offer for eye sight. Carrots are rich in vitamin A, which is the vitamin required for proper eye sight.

Carrots also have a high lutene content which is an antioxidant. Foods that have high lutene content have been shown to increase pigment density in the macula. In short…The higher the pigment density the more your eye is protected and the less chance you'll have vision issues which lead to headaches.

Tip 15.

Do not look at the sun directly. This may seem like a "no-brainer" but you would be surprised at what we see as causes for headaches for people that work outside on a daily basis. This is especially true for the hours between 7 a.m. in the morning and 4 p.m. in the evening. If you are going to be outside during this time or driving, be sure to shield your eyes in some manner.

Tip 16.

Wear sunglasses. Do it. Even in the winter. You must protect your eyes. Sunglasses are the best protection that you can give your eyes when you go out in the sun. The sun beats down ultra violet and other harmful radiations. Your eyes need protection from these radiations because they can cause serious damage to your eyes when they are directly exposed. Below are some tips for choosing sunglasses:

- The sunglasses must cover the *entire* region of your eyes completely.
- Sunglasses lenses may be of any color that you like, but make sure that they guard your eyes against ultra violet radiations.
- Choose lenses that are easy to clean and are easy to keep free from dust and smudges.
- The best way to choose your sunglasses is to put them on and stare at your face in a mirror. If you can see your eyes in the mirror, then the glasses are *not* going to protect your eyes from sunlight.

Tip 17.

Do not work continuously on your computer for more than half an hour. This, in fact, is a very relative concept because some people tire faster than others when working on the computer. Computer screens emit radiation, so the less time in front of the computer, the better.

If your eyes give you signs that they have had enough, *take the cue*. Most people, however, get used to working on the computer and ignore these signs. The best thing you can do is make it a point to give your eyes *and mind* break at least every half hour of working on the computer.

The best way to give your eyes a rest while doing computer work is to stare at a *distant object*. You can also try *massaging* your eyes gently. The following is a great method for massaging your eyes:

- When you massage your eyes take care to use only the soft balls of your fingers. Do not use your finger tips because your nails could give you scratches.

- The best fingers to massage your eyes with are the three middle fingers, which are the fingers between your thumb and the little finger.

- Place the balls of your fingers on your eyebrows and gently press down. Please remember to be gentle--we are not talking about a major massage therapy here.

- Now let your fingers roll down around your eyes making gentle circling movements. The motion should start from the eyebrows and end at the corners of the eyes near the nose bridge.

- Repeat this two or three times and you can feel your eye muscles relax.

- It is a good idea to this at least five or six times a day if you are working at something that gives a lot of strain to your eyes.

Remember that your eyes are unlike any other part of your body so you must take very good care of them.

Tip 18.

Do not watch television while laying down. It forces your neck into an undesirable position and likely will cause muscle tension and nerve pressure as well vascular compression. The best position to watch television is sitting and your eyes should preferably be at the level of the television screen.

Tip 19.

Do not sit too close to your television set. Take care to sit a considerable distance from the screen. This will make it easier for your eyes to focus on the images that flash across your TV screen. It is also less harmful for your eyes. The ideal distance from your TV set is around five feet or more.

Tip 20.

Do not watch television in the dark. Make sure that the room in which your television or computer is located in is properly lit. Watching television or working on the computer in the dark unnecessarily strains your eyes. Make sure to always turn on a lamp or overhead light.

Tip 21.

Blink. Try to *blink* deliberately while working on the computer. There is an increased tendency to stare without blinking at the monitor especially when you are involved in intense work or playing an exciting game. In such cases, you should make a conscious effort to blink your eyes.

If you do not blink, your eyes will become dry and hurt, and this will ultimately precipitate into a headache. Blinking allows your eyelids wash your eyeballs with the tear secretions. Your eyeballs must stay moist so always remember to *blink* your eyes even if you are deeply engrossed in something interesting.

Tip 22.

***Do breathing* exercises.** This will help you breathe better and release toxins from your brain. The human body takes in a lot of toxic substances, both through the air and through food and drink you consume. Apart from this, various toxins are also released in the body as a result of the various processes that are going on. These toxins have to be released on a continuous basis or else they will accumulate in the body with serious results.

One of the best ways of releasing these toxins is through exhaling while breathing. One unknown fact is most of us *do not breathe properly.* With each breath that we take, we take in oxygen. This oxygen is carried by the blood to every cell of the body and every cell must indeed get enough oxygen, not just to survive, but to remain healthy.

So it is imperative that we make an honest attempt to breathe properly. The following is a great example of how to do proper breathing exercises which will allow your brain to fill with oxygen and to push out those toxins:

- Breathe in unpolluted air. The time best for breathing exercises is early in the morning when the air is comparatively unpolluted.

- Sit comfortably so that there is no strain to any part of your body. It is not imperative that you close your eyes, but I have always noticed that the exercise works better when the eyes are closed.

- When you are ready, breathe in deeply and slowly, and feel the fresh air filling up your lungs until it just can't take any more. Conjure up images of the air encircling throughout your body and reaching every cell, literally bathing it with oxygen. Of course, it doesn't happen that way, but the image helps a lot. Then hold your breath for a few seconds, and then very slowly exhale letting out all that foul air. *Note: The longer you hold the air in your lungs, and the longer you take to exhale, the better.*

- Once again, conjure up an image of all the toxins being released from your body. Every cell has now become free of the burden it was carrying. Now pause for a second or two, and again breathe in deeply and slowly letting your lungs fill up with all that good, clean, rejuvenating air. Repeat this exercise at least ten times. Also be sure to take your time, taking care not to rush through it.

When you have completed the above you are now ready for the second part of the breathing exercise:

- Again sit with your eyes closed, but this time, keep your right nostril closed with the help of your right index-finger. Now breathe in deeply and slowly through your left nostril keeping the right nostril closed. When you have held air for a second or two, release your right nostril and breathe out through it.

- While you are breathing out conjure up an image of all the toxins being released form your head and the brain especially. As you breathe in, conjure up images of the clean air circulating though out your brain freeing it of all the worries and trouble and lightening it. *Note: Again, that the longer you hold the air in your lungs, and the longer you take to exhale, the better.*

- Repeat this exercise with the left nostril closed and in this way alternate between the nostrils at least ten times. The entire breathing exercise should take less than ten minutes.

Tip 23.

Be careful of pillow size. Use a pillow that is not too thick or too thin to rest your head. If the pillow that you are using is does not fit you correctly, you will be straining you neck muscles when you are asleep. If the neck muscles stay taught for too long, they will become stiff and this often precipitates as a headache. When you are laying flat on your back or on either side, your posture should be as though you are standing straight up. That is, your head should not be flexed forward or extended back when you are on your back and should not be tilted to the left or right when you are on your side.

Tip 24.

Find out if you have any allergies. Allergies can cause headaches. Some of us are allergic to specific substances that can trigger the onset of a headache. It may be certain odors or it might be a certain flavors. Each time you get a headache, try and find out if there is a commonality which may have triggered it. This contributing factor may indeed be an allergy.

Tip 25.

Keep your hair dry. Make sure you *dry* your hair and head well after a shower. It is best to use a towel for drying. The problem with leaving your hair wet is that water can seep in through the scalp of your head, which in turn can cause a headache to come on. This is a highly debated cause of headaches.

Tip 26.

Do not blow dry your hair. The heat from the dryer is actually harmful and can cause damage to the pores on your head. This heat can onset a headache rapidly.

Tip 27.

If you must blow dry your hair, keep the dryer well away from your head. If you must use a dryer, use it only on long hair. Never use it to blow dry short hair. Not only is the heat harmful to your head and a headache inducer, but the drone of the dryer can also cause a headache.

Tip 28.

Protect your head from the sun. The sun has many benefits as far as health is concerned, but if you expose yourself directly to the sun, you are likely to end up with a headache.

The heat from the sun can bring about vascular changes and alter the delicate balance of the various fluids inside the brain. This, in all likelihood, will precipitate as a whale of a headache. That is why it is imperative that you protect your head with a cap or a hat when you have to go out in the sun.

Tip 29.

Stay out of the rain. It is not good idea to let rain fall directly on your head. Rain water may be refreshing but in can result in a headache. Rain water contains pollutants. This is especially true for the first rains of the season. Early rainwater will contain a concentration of pollutants and this itself, may result in a lot of diseases. If you get wet in the rain, make it a point to dry your hair and head as soon as you can.

Tip 30.

Avoid inhaling polluting gases. Automobile fumes and second-hand smoke are the most common fumes people are exposed to daily. Many of the gases let out by automobiles and other exhaust pipes are highly toxic and can cause a headache. The second-hand smoke that you inhale from your neighbor's cigarette can also cause a headache. This is especially true if you are a non-smoker and not used to the smell smoke. Both of these common gases are triggers to headaches.

Tip 31.

Do not pull your hair up too tight. Some people, especially women, tie up their hair in very tight ponytails, buns or braids. When your hair is pulled back too tightly for too long, it will put a lot of tension on your scalp causing pain and resulting in a headache.

Tip 32.

Realize that stress may be the cause. Many of us carry the weight of the world on our shoulders. This can cause constant tension in our bodies, especially the neck and trap muscles. Try to keep your mind free from worries. Listening to music or taking a nap is a good way to clear the mind. The less you worry, the less tension you have, the less likely you will develop a headache. This may seem like a "no brainer" but you would be surprised how many people come in with headaches and don't make the connection.

Tip 33.

Relax. If you feel stressed take a warm bath, listen to soothing music or burn a scented candle. These are all ways to help relax your body and to release tension in the muscles that bring on headaches.

Tip 34.

Sleep. Getting a good night of sleep is a *necessity* for keeping headaches at bay. Sleeping is one activity in which *everyone* must do. However, with today's technology and the fast pace in which we all live, getting the required quantity and quality of sleep we need is becoming harder and harder.

The National Sleep Foundation reports (2002) that America is on the verge of a poor sleep epidemic, characterized by the following eye-opening statistics:

- 64% of American adults get less than the eight hours of sleep that experts recommend is required to maintain optimal physical, mental, and emotional health.
- One-third of the US population says they get less sleep now than they did five years ago.
- One-half of Americans have experienced insomnia (sleeplessness).
- Drowsiness due to a lack of a proper night of sleep interferes with the daily activities of 37 percent of all adults.

You need peace and quiet to get enough sleep and you should take care to see that there are no physical disturbances. Turn the ring tone of your telephone to the lowest possible volume. Do not worry about important calls--if the call is so important, then the caller will call back again. Try to cut out other disturbances by wearing ear muffs or eye blinds. *Do not read in bed before you sleep.* In all likelihood, you will drift off to sleep with the lights on, and after sometime, the same light will wake you up.

Tip 35.

Do not oversleep. Oversleeping is just as bad as not getting enough sleep. If you sleep too much or for too long, you may wake up with a very woozy feeling and that will most likely turn into a headache. Our body tells us when it has had enough sleep. Listen to the cue and get up. Do not succumb to the temptation to just lie in bed.

Tip 36.

Get the right amount of sleep for you. Studies have shown that eight hours is the requirement for most healthy adults. However, not every person needs this requirement, and some people need more. Babies and young children require more sleep to nurture their growing bodies and older individuals need more to rest their aging bodies. Young adults tend to function better with a little less than the 8 hours but, as the saying goes—it eventually catches up with them later on in life. Whichever the case, be sure to examine your daily schedule to ensure that you will be able to get the right amount of sleep. Try to cut out television and other non-necessary activities.

Tip 37.

Stay away from sedatives. However easy they make it, sedatives are not a solution to your sleep problems. Many of them are addictive and eventually the medicine will stop working for you. Sedatives also affect the time that you wake up. You may get the amount of sleep needed when you take them, but the chances are rare that you will wake up refreshed.

Tip 38.

Avoid aspirin. If you take aspirin for every headache you have, your body will become dependent on needing it to take your headache away. We all know that some headaches go away by themselves. Be as patient as you possible can and try to wait the headache out. Do not make your body dependent on aspirin.

Tip 39.

Massage your temples. Massaging your temples gently stimulates the circulation of blood and relaxes the muscles of the forehead and temples. This itself soothes a person and provides relief from headaches.

Tip 40.

Touch therapy. This is a new technique that is just becoming known as a cure for headaches. Many studies have been done in this area, but experts have been unable to identify exactly how touch therapy can help in healing. The best possible explanation is that our bodies are in fact tuned to respond to the touches of others.

When we were babies, our mother's touch was perhaps the most reassuring thing in the world. In fact, experts are baffled by the way new born babies are able to distinguish their own mother's touch from the touch of a stranger.

As we grow older, we delight in the encouraging pats and caresses of our parents and loved ones. Even in our social lives there is a lot of touching going on--this is probably why people use hugs, high-fives and hand-shakes as exchanges of warmth.

When you are ill and miserable, the touch of another person, especially if it is a person who really cares for you can relieve you of your pain. The gentle touch of a loved one is more healing to the body and mind than we know and this touch can stop a headache in its tracks.

Tip 41.

Massage key points of your body. These areas include the nape of your neck, the shoulder and neck muscles, and the muscles at the web between your thumb and the rest of your fingers.

The entire nervous system, the blood vessels, the skeletal and muscular systems are all interconnected. So if you can identify certain nodal points of the body and apply the right pressure there, you can indeed get relief from a headache. This is the basic philosophy of the principle of acupressure. Just be careful to apply the right amount of pressure. Too much pressure can be damaging to the tissue. Pressure that is not adequate enough may not have the desired effect.

Tip 42.

Do not wash your hair in hot water. This can trigger a lot of vascular changes that can do more harm than good. Though a hot bath may be stimulating to your body, it is not the best thing that you can give your head.

Take a steam bath if you want to, but try to keep your head above the steamy fumes. Cold water is best for your head, *so keep it that way*. By cold water, we are not referring to chilled water.

Tip 43.

Watch out for smells. The fragrances of some perfumes and room fresheners are major causes of headaches. This includes all smells, not only the ones you use on your own body. It can be a perfume that your neighbor is wearing. So if the person you are sitting by is wearing a smell that does not agree with you and you feel that your head is getting woozy, try to move to a safe distance. Avoiding these smells quickly can stop a headache.

Tip 44.

Avoid incense smoke. Incense smoke is not good for you. It contains a lot of alkaloids and the inhalation of these can spark changes in the internal mechanism. Do not take the risk.

Tip 45.

Regulate noise. Too much noise is bad for you. In fact, sound pollution is one of the major causes that headaches have become so prevalent.

Contrary to popular belief, sound pollution is not only caused by machines and automobiles. A journey down the street during the rush hour is enough to give any body a headache, but apart from that, blaring music can and does a lot of harm as well.

Take care to lower the volume if you want to listen to music. If you want to play music in order to soothe your nerves and you are playing loud music, it will have just the opposite effect. Your blood pressure will actually go up and your adrenalin levels will increase. The best thing that you can do is avoid all sources of loud noises.

Tip 46.

Use ear plugs. If you are moving into a loud sound zone, use ear plugs, ear muffs or thick wads of cotton to reduce the sound level. Most grocery stores and convenience stores carry sound-reducing and sound-blocking earplugs, many of which are not noticeable.

Tip 47.

Try steam inhalation. This is especially true for those who have a sinus problem. Steam inhalation is an excellent way of clearing the sinus spaces in your face and head. If you have an infection, steam inhalation can relieve the pressure and be very soothing.

However, be very careful about you eyes. Remember that it is not advisable to expose your eyes to steam, so take care to protect your eyes when you are inhaling steam.

Also, be careful about the temperature of the steam. You just need fairly hot water, not scorching hot or sizzling vapors of water. The object is not to scald your skin, but to send some warm vapors up your nose. In fact, steam inhalation is one of the most recommended therapies for people who get sinus related headaches.

The point that you should keep in mind is that the faster you inhale steam once a headache ensues, the better. If you wait for long hours before you inhale, you are going to have to inhale longer and at shorter intervals for the inhalation to have any effect on the headache.

Tip 48.

Inhale menthol vapors. This can be a great source of relief. Menthol vapors help by clearing and opening your sinuses. Try dissolving a menthol balm or ointment in hot water and inhaling the steam. This will help clean out the sinus cavities and relieve headache pain.

Tip 49.

Quit smoking. Just do it. Smoking can affect your head in very harmful ways. In fact, smoking affects the functioning of *every* part of your body. When you smoke, you actually submit your body, and the various mechanisms that go on in it, to the power of the very strong alkaloid *nicotine.* So if you can quit smoking by all means do. It will help you live a better life and can contribute much towards eliminating your headaches.

There are many things that are identified with substance abuse. Alcohol is one of them, narcotic drugs are another, and tobacco is in no way to be left behind. The problem, or let us say that the similarity among all these substances, is that once one gets used to them, breaking away is not easy. In fact, if your headache goes away when you start smoking a cigarette, it means that your body has already become dependent on nicotine. In that case, your headache may be a withdrawal symptom.

Contrary to popular belief, it is not the fear of deprivation of the pleasantly high feeling that drives the person to use the substance again and again so that it is used, misused and eventually abused. The person returns for his or her daily fix because of certain altered conditions in the body. These substances are indeed very potent and they affect certain specific spots or centers of the brain.

The brain quickly gets used to these alterations and then before we know it, these centers of the brain cannot do without the daily dose of the substance. The brain did not ask for the substance in the first place, but we gave them to it. When we experience that pleasantly high feeling, we do not bother about the changes that are taking place within.

It is common knowledge that the entire processes carried about in the brain are maintained by a delicate balance of the various chemical located there. Once we start using substances like tobacco, narcotics and alcohol, the balance of these chemicals get altered.

The body, as I mentioned earlier is a self-adjusting machine, and so this new chemical balance is established and it takes no time for the brain cells to get adjusted to the new balance. Then, when the brain cells do not get what is required to maintain the new balance, things go haywire.

However, this new balance is not the real or natural balance, it is something that has to be artificially supported. When that daily or timely dose of nicotine does not get to the brain, the new balance gets upset and a headache may occur.

Tip 50.

Do not drink coffee. Just like with nicotine, the caffeine in coffee is addictive. If you have the habit of drinking a cup of coffee at a fixed time every day, you will in all likelihood end up with a headache if your body does not get that required dose of coffee.

The point to ponder about is this: *Why do you have to make your body dependent on external substances when it can function very well without these substances?*

Tip 51.

Water. Water. Water. Drink plenty of water. Water is the most important substance that your body needs. If you are not drinking enough water, you may suffer from a dehydration headache. For a person to remain healthy, he or she must drink at least ten glasses of water a day. As a matter of fact, it is recommended that a person drink half of their weight in ounces of water each day. This means that a 200 lb person should drink 100 ounces of water each day. If your intake of water is less than this then by all means drink more water.

The more water you drink, the better you will feel. If you do not drink enough water, the water balance of the body will be completely disrupted. Make no mistake about this--the major content of all the cells in your body is indeed water. When your body does not get enough water, it will end up dehydrated. This will invariably result in a headache.

Tip 52.

Do not let water get into your ears. This is especially true of pool water. In most pools, chemicals are added to the water to keep it clean and disinfected. These chemicals however are not the best thing for your body. So it is always advisable to cover your head with some protective material.

If water does go into your ears, try and get it out as soon as you can. Otherwise, you may develop a ringing sensation in your ears, which is next door to a headache. The best way to get rid of the water in your ear is to pour in a little more water and then tilt you head to the side of the ear that has water in it. This action should allow the water in your ear to drain out.

Tip 53.

Cool your eye muscles with slices of cucumber. Cucumbers hydrate the skin around the eye and help eliminate inflammation, which in turn will allow the muscle of the eye to relax.

This is a 100% natural method of cooling your eyes and you will be surprised at how refreshed you feel when you remove those slices after a couple of minutes.

Tip 54.

Do eye exercises. Eye exercises allow you to strengthen the musculature of the eye which will help to avoid ocular fatigue. The following is a great example of how to do eye strengthening exercises:

1. Stare straight ahead of you preferably at a distant object.

2. Close your eyes and let any glimmers of light fade away.

3. Now open your eyes and move your eye balls to the extreme top of your eye sockets and keep them there for a few seconds.

4. Now move them down to the extreme bottom and keep them

there for a few seconds.

5. Next, move them to the extreme left.

6. Then bring them to the extreme right.

7. Finally focus your eye on your nose and hold, then slowly focus on the distant object again.

8. Repeat this exercise three or four times a day.

By strengthening the eye musculature you reduce the likelihood of eye fatigue which is a serious causation of headaches.

Tip 55.

Use soothing face masks. Face masks are a wonderful way of de-stressing yourself. Many grocery stores and beauty supply stores carry them.

You can make your own face mask at home using things that are 100% safe on your skin. One of the best face masks that I have come across, that is equally effective for a sinus headache as well as a tension headache, is a curd face pack.

Chill curd in the refrigerator for a few minutes. If you do not have curd, yogurt will work. Apply a thin coating of this curd or yogurt on your forehead and on the region around your eyes. Be careful to see that it does not get into your eyes. When you feel that the first coat has dried up apply one more coat. Then lie down with your face up for five to ten minutes. This process will help to relieve tension in your face and eye musculature and help to diminish the likelihood of a headache.

Tip 56.

De-stress. If you are a tension headache sufferer, this is a must. Remember, tension headaches happen when the muscles in your neck and head get tight due to a stressor. De-stressing when a headache comes on will prevent the headache from becoming full-blown.

A great way to de-stress is through meditation. This brings with it peace of mind as we learn to observe our surroundings. We become one with our surroundings and it helps us to focus our mental energy on one thing at a time. The human mind is a virtual power house of energy, but often this energy goes un-channeled or untapped. Through the process of meditation, we can harness this energy and use it for constructive purposes.

In the initial stages you may find your mind drifting, but gradually you will learn to focus more and more. The idea behind meditation is not to cut out all the forces around, you but to become one with them.

I have seen people plug their ears with cotton to shut out sounds. However, this is not the purpose that we wish to achieve. On the contrary, we should focus on the sounds around us.

Be aware of the sounds and listen to them. First, listen to the bigger sounds around you like the traffic or machines or even loud music from your neighbor's apartment.

Then listen to the softer sounds like the drone of the refrigerator, or the A/C. Then bring your attention to the sound of your own breathing. If you can actually hear yourself breathing, then you have arrived and this is what you have to keep doing.

Try to focus on the here and now, and not on tomorrow or yesterday. After all, we all live in today and not in the yesterdays and tomorrows!

The following technique for meditation and is a good way to de-stress and get your mind and body in the right place:

The Mind Settling Procedure:

1. Sit comfortably in silence with your eyes closed for 30 seconds.

2. Perform a brief body massage. (Some meditation traditions recommend that the massage be executed slightly differently for men and women, and I would like to describe these recommendations here. To be frank with you, I am not clear as to why these gender-related differences exist, or if the

need for the differences is real).

3. The massage for both men and women begins by gently pressing the hands against the face, then upward on the top of the head, back down the neck, and towards the heart. (By the way, all massage elements move towards, and finish at the heart).

4. Men continue by gently using the left hand to press and massage, first the right hand, and then up the arm, and back down towards the heart. Again, this is all done with the left hand.

5. Women do the same, but they begin by massaging the left hand and arm (back toward the heart) with the right hand. Then both men and women switch arms and massage the other hand and arm, again, back toward the heart.

6. Men continue by massaging the right foot and leg, upward toward the heart. This is done by pressing with both hands gently. Then, massage the left foot and leg, again, upward toward the heart. Women do the same, but they begin with the left foot and leg, upward toward the heart, before repeating the process for the right foot and leg. This is best done with the eyes closed. The total time for the massage is about a minute.

7. While sitting comfortably with the back straight, perform a breathing technique that is called *pranayama (feel free to "Google" this for a video on how to do it).* Begin with 10 seconds of fast pranayama. This is done using very short, gentle breaths, closing one nostril at a time after each outward and inward breath.

8. Next, close the nostrils (one at a time) with the thumb and the middle fingers (alternately) of one hand. Men use their right hand to do this while women use their left. This is best done with the eyes closed. The procedure should be effortless and easy, and if someone is experiencing any problems like dizziness or hyperventilation, it is being performed incorrectly

and its practice should be discontinued until getting personal instructions in this technique.

9. While sitting comfortably with the back straight, perform 9 to 10 minutes of slow pranayama. This is done similarly as with the fast pranayama, but using normal breaths (not short or long ones), closing one nostril at a time after each outward and inward breath. Be sure to complete both the outward and inward breath before switching nostrils. On exhaling, let the breath flow out naturally, not forcing it. The inhaling breath should take about half the time as the exhaling breath.

10. Keeping your eyes closed, hold your breath after inhaling for a brief moment (a second or two) while alternatively closing the other nostril with the other finger, and prepare to exhale. The entire procedure should be effortless and gentle. If you feel you need more air, simply take deeper breaths, but do not hyperventilate. You should be breathing normally, just alternating nostrils after exhaling and inhaling.

11. Sit quietly and comfortably for 5 minutes with the eyes closed.

Tip 57.

Listen to soft music. This helps ease your mind, which in turn, helps to relax muscles preventing tension and headaches. Do this preferably without earphones.

Tip 58.

Practice yoga. It sounds simple, but it really does work. Tension that is caused by forward head posture and slumping forward can be relieved through many different yoga poses.

Tip 59.

Pray. No matter what your religion, prayer allows you to release worries and anxieties and calms your mind. Prayer is an excellent way of de-stressing yourself. There are plenty of studies out there to actually back up the relaxing effects of prayer.

Tip 60.

Stop drinking alcohol. Reduce your alcohol consumption to only 2 – 3 glasses per week. If headaches persist, try to quit completely. Alcohol is a known trigger for migraine headaches, not to mention the dehydration headache it can cause, commonly known as a hangover. Just drink water instead. This may not be near as fun, but a million times the health.

Tip 61.

Avoid hangovers. If you must consume alcohol, do not drink to excess, as to avoid a hangover. The following tips can help you avoid a hangover headache.

- Since a hangover headache is usually the result of dehydration, if you increase your intake of water, you can keep a hangover headache at bay. Always stay fully hydrated by the drinking 10 glasses of water per day so you do not start out with a water deficit.

- When drinking mixed drinks, dilute your drink with water instead of soda. The more water you take in, the better.

- Never start drinking on an empty stomach. Eat something! Also, munch on snacks while you are drinking.

- Drink a glass of milk one or two hours before you leave for the party. This will help with the amount of alcohol your body will absorb and deplete of water.

- For every ounce of alcohol that you consume, make it a point to consume a glass of plain water. This will help replace the amount of water that is depleted from the alcohol in your body.

Tip 62.

Avoid frustration. Easier said than done, I know, but frustration can easily bring on a tension headache. Whether it is caused by work, taking care of the kids, or other factors, when you feel yourself loosing control, take a step back and take 10 deep breaths. This will calm you and reduce the muscle tension build up.

Tip 63.

Be careful with color choices. The colors around you can have an impact on the way your mind works. This is especially true when it comes to the rooms you spend most of your time in.

> Red and orange are *not* the most suitable colors for your bedroom and the living room--the two rooms that people tend to spend the majority of their time. It is better to go for light pastel shades or dark soothing colors like blues and greens.

Tip 64.

Get your teeth checked. Bad teeth can cause headaches. If you have a tooth infection that is left untreated, there is a very good chance that the pain will go on to the rest of your head. If the bad tooth is in the upper jaw bone, you have a greater chance of getting a headache.

Never take a bad tooth lightly. Get the help of your dentist as soon as you feel that there is something wrong with your teeth. If you let it go, you are facing a high risk of developing a headache that just won't go away.

Tip 65.

Focus on your posture. The wrong sitting posture can result in a headache. If you do not sit properly when you are working, you could cause the muscles of your neck and shoulders to cramp. Remember that if the muscles of you neck are cramped, it will result in a headache. The following will help you to get the correct posture:

- Do not slouch in your chair. Try to sit as erect as possible with your feet planted on the floor.

- Do not cross your legs at the knees or ankles.
- Square your shoulders. Do not allow them to roll forward.
- Make sure your head is looking straight and your monitor is at eye level. Your head should not be tilted to the left or right and it should not be flexed forward.
- Instead of bending your head forward, try to hold whatever you have to do up so that your neck is straight.

If you find you continue to have bad posture, you may consider buying a lumbar support pad, a doughnut pillow or other devices designed to make you sit correctly. These are available in office stores and medical supply stores.

Tip 66.

Wash out the hair gel. Remove hair gel before going to bed. Hair gel may give you that great look, but it also seals off the pores in your scalp. This prevents the skin on your head from breathing. Hair gel also contains a fair amount of chemicals that are not good for your body and can trigger headaches. These chemicals may seep through the pores or be inhaled while you are sleeping. Hair gels are likely to also have mild perfumes that also trigger migraines.

Tip 67.

Avoid aerosols. Aerosols are used in everything from hairspray to spray paint and contain harmful chemicals that are not found in nature. When these chemicals are inhaled, they prohibit oxygen from getting to the brain, causing dizziness, light-headedness and headaches.

Tip 68.

If you wear glasses or contacts, get your eyes checked periodically. The wrong prescription, whether it be too strong or too weak, can cause your eyes to work harder to compensate for the blurry vision. This causes fatigue of the ocular musculature and may result in frequent headaches. Once you develop a defect with your vision, it is a very good idea to get yourself tested at least once every six months.

Tip 69.

If you have perfect vision, get your eyes checked periodically. Most vision defects are hereditary, so if one of your parents started using glasses at an early age, there is 25% chance that you might have the same problem at some point in your life as well.

Tip 70.

Never shake your head violently. You may want to refrain from riding fast rollercoasters, or even driving on unfinished roads. This causes the neck muscles to become tight and may result in a tension headache.

Tip 71.

Do shake your head gently if you suspect a sinus headache. A gentle shake of your head however, can tell you if you do have a sinus infection. If you move your head even slightly, the pain will increase and this is a good method of deciding whether the headache is actually due to a sinus infection. One a sinus headache is determined avoid any shaking of the head.

Tip 72.

Bend over if you suspect a sinus headache. The moment you lower your head you will feel as if there is something heavy inside your head. This is a shift in the fluid of your sinuses. This is an indicator that there may be a sinus infection present. If doing so leads you to discover you have a sinus infection, refrain from bending over until the infection clears.

Tip 73.

Keep calm. Anger and irritation are major causes of headaches. This is most likely due to the muscle tension and jaw clenching that occurs when anger sweeps over us. It is best to walk away from someone that is irritating you then to allow them to be the cause of your headache.

Tip 74.

Avoid stuffy rooms. Stuffy rooms occur when there is not enough air circulating in the room. If the room smells musty too, it is a good idea to get out of the room or open all the windows and doors and let the fresh air come in. Pollutants in uncirculated rooms can trigger a headache.

Tip 75.

Do not sleep in rooms without proper ventilation. Make sure that clean air is circulating in the room and you are not breathing in polluted air. Sleeping in a room that is not properly ventilated may cause you to wake up unrested due to lack of good oxygen, and also with a headache. Even if the A/C is turned on, try to also turn on the fan to circulate the air.

Tip 76.

Soothe a sore head. Dipping a cotton ball in iced water and applying it to your forehead will help ease the sore feeling. Another way is to apply an ice pack to your forehead. Remember, the objective is to cool your head not freeze it, so only leave it on 10-15 minutes.

Tip 77.

Try not to cry. I know that sometimes there are situations where crying is unavoidable, but if you are a crier, note that crying can lead to a headache. Crying from stress or sadness reduces the body's hormone levels which often causes a headache to ensue.

If you feel you might start crying, try breathing deeply, or try to lie down. Some situations are unavoidable, but some, like sad movies, are easy to avoid.

Tip 78.

Do not skip meals. Hunger is the worst enemy of a person who is prone to migraine attacks. When you miss meals or have meals at times other than normal, you are actually depriving your body of the much needed energy.

The body will seek out alternative measures and will start working on fat reserves. The fats cannot be easily converted to sugars, which the body desperately needs. So when the body does not get what it wants, the cells get deprived of energy and this manifests itself in the form of a headache. It is important to eat at fixed times throughout the day.

Tip 79.

Blow your nose. Blowing your nose helps to get rid of the mucus that accumulates in the sinuses. It is better if you can blow your nose after a steam inhalation. This will help prevent the onset of sinusitis and headaches due to sinus issues.

Tip 80.

Do a water rinse in your nose. This is a very effective way of clearing your sinuses and saving your self from a bout of dust allergy as well. All you have to do is cup your hand and hold a little bit of water in it. Dip you nose in and inhale the water very gently.

The water must only ascend the passage of your nose and must not go any further. You can control the ascent of the water by controlling your breath. After this, breathe out and let the water out. Repeat this process a couple of times. You might snort the first two or three times, but after that you will soon get the hang of it.

Tip 81

Stay away from dust. If you have an allergic condition like a dust allergy, try to stay away from dust. Dust can trigger the onset of a sinus infection. Make sure you change your air filters regularly, and consider buying special filters for people with dust allergies. If you find it impossible to stay away from dust, at least wear a mask. This will help with the amount of dust you inhale.

Tip 82.

Do not sleep on your stomach. Sleeping on your stomach causes you to turn your head to breath. This causes your spine to rotate and the muscles in your neck to be pulled tight. This position can also cause the vascular system in your neck to be compromised.

Tip 83.

Avoid MSG, caffeine and aspartame. Foods containing MSG (monosodium glutamate), caffeine and aspartame (which is a common artificial sweetener) are known causes for migraines. These substances are found in thousands of foods and drinks. Avoid them as much as possible.

Tip 84.

Do not eat fermented and pickled food. These foods have high levels of tyramine, which is a natural food chemical that affects signals along the pain nerve endings. They can be harmful to you, especially if you suffer from frequent headaches.

Tip 85.

Know your birth control side effects. Contraceptive pills can trigger headaches because they actually interfere with the hormonal functioning of the body.

Tip 86.

Maintain a headache diary. I know that the idea might sound strange, but do it. You should monitor the foods and beverages you ingest, weather conditions, stresses and menstrual cycles.

Try to identify the causes that lead to the headache or, in other words, the causes that trigger of the headache. Find out how often and how frequent the headaches are, and whether they are related to any external condition like the weather or travel. It is really not very difficult to do this.

This exercise will help the person find out if there are definite causes and what is to be avoided in order to prevent the onset of a headache.

Tip 87.

See a doctor. Many people feel uneasy about going to a doctor with something as insignificant as a headache. However, there is nothing *really* insignificant about a headache.

It is one of the most maddening things in the world. Every year the nation loses millions of dollars worth of productive days because good workers go down with headaches.

There is nothing to feel bad about consulting a doctor about a headache. In fact, many practitioners do a thriving business by setting up headache clinics. If you have a headache diary, like the one we mentioned in the above point, it would be very useful to your doctor in reaching a good diagnosis.

Let me stress this, it is *fine* to tell you doctor that you do not want over to be on over the counter medication or any other medications for that matter.

Your doctor works for you, and a good one will give you alternatives for medication if requested.

Give your doctor a complete list of the all the medicines that you consume. You have to remember that some of these medicines might be altering your vascular system leading to a headache. The medicines that you need to take particular note of, are birth control pills, medicines for blood pressure, and any hormone supplements.

Tip 88.

Do not wear restricted clothing. Dress suitable when you are indoors as well as outdoors. Your choice of what to wear must be in complete harmony with the weather conditions and the temperature around you.

You have to understand that too much is just as bad as too little. If you wrap yourself up tightly all the time, you are in fact restricting the flow of blood to certain parts of the body. As we know, restriction of blood flow can cause headaches to arise.

Ties and scarves must be avoided as much as possible and if you have to wear these, try to keep them as loose as possible.

Tip 89.

Let your body adjust to time changes. While traveling, it is very important to allow your body adequate rest. For example, if you are flying across the International Date Line, there is every chance that you will experience what is popularly known as the jet lag. Give you body time to adjust to such uncommon things.

Try your best to get the sleep that your body needs while you are traveling. Do not bury your nose in a book or watch a movie,
SLEEP!

Tip 90.

Use acupressure. Know your sinus points and use the acupressure method to treat your self and rid yourself of the pain.

The absolute best thing about the acupressure method is that it has *no* side effects. It is something that you can do completely on your own and if you are doing it properly, you can get almost instant relief. I have described the steps in detail in the points that follow, try doing these and I promise you, you will be glad that you did:

1. Get a clear idea of where your sinuses really are. For this, I

recommend that you lie down on a flat surface preferably without the support of a pillow.

2. Next, run your fingers gently over your face, taking note of the various rises and falls.

3. Now let your fingers linger in the portion above your eyes but just below the eyebrow.

4. Feel the bone and let you fingers sense out a notch in that bone. This space extends from there towards the nasal bone. This is your first sinus point.

5. Now let your fingers trail down further until they reach the depressions on both sides of the nose halfway between the eyes and your mouth. This is your second sinus point.

6. Now apply pressure to these sinus points. You must be careful when you do this. Please take care to use only the soft balls of your fingers and not the tips, which may have long nails.

7. Now apply pressure gently. You might experience a particular pricking sensation as you do.

8. If it hurts, you may stop immediately.

9. If there is no pain, continue applying more and more pressure as long as you can tolerate it.

10. Then, gently let go and lie there fore a minute experiencing the pain fading away.

11. Repeat this with the second sinus point.

12. Keep in mind that if your sinuses are infected, these regions will be slightly swollen.

Tip 91.

Exercise. Do it. Exercise is a good way to prevent headaches. It is a wonderful way of increasing the blood flow to the various organs and parts of your body. So if you can develop a regular exercise pattern, you will in fact be ensuring a better blood circulation and proper supply of oxygen to the various cells of the body.

Tip 92.

Stretch. Elongating your muscles helps to avoid cramping and muscle tightness. Never let cramps set in. If you feel that you have been in a position for too long, stretch yourself. Rub your hands and feet and the muscles of your neck to boost up the circulation.

Tip 93.

Do this specific technique when a tension headache comes on. This is an exercise that is usually done by an expert, but I assure you that it is perfectly safe to do it on your own too.

1. Place your right hand on the top of your head or let it rest on your forehead.

2. Now gently turn your head towards the right. This will clear the left side of your neck so that your left hand can have easy access to it.

3. Now place the palm of your left hand on the back of your neck and let your fingers try to sense out any muscle that is particularly taut.

4. For this, all you have to do is let your fingers creep along your neck like the legs of a spider but with a little more force.

5. When you have found a tight muscle, gently apply pressure on it using the soft balls of your fingers.

6. As you apply pressure, breathe in air and hold the air for ten to

twenty seconds.

7. As you hold the air, the application of pressure must continue.

8. Concentrate on the releasing of the tension of that muscle.

9. Convince your mind that all the toxins that were pent up in that muscle have now been released.

10. When you feel that the muscle has relaxed, release your grip and at the same time breathe out through your mouth, feeling that all the toxins have been released from your body.

11. Repeat the exercise on the same side of your neck and try to find another muscle.

12. In this way continue till all the muscles on the left side are done.

13. Now repeat this exercise with right side of your neck and using your right hand this time.

Tip 94.

Measure your migraine. Your migraine can be measure in terms of the following criteria:

- Frequency: How often do you get the migraine? Knowing how often a migraine occurs will help to determine if there is a hormonal component to the headache.

- Intensity: How severe is the pain? You can measure this yourself using a 5-point scale. Zero stands for no pain at all, while 5 means that you have the worst pain that you have ever had.

- Duration: How long does the pain last? Does it go away by itself or you have to get a deep sleep before you get any relief.

- Medication: Do you have to take any medicines before you get any relief from it, and if you have to do how many medicines do you take and in what quantity?

This measuring of your migraine should also be kept in your headache journal. This information will help with the determination of diagnosis and treatment.

Tip 95.

Take a warm shower. You have to understand that a tension headache comes purely from tight cervical and neck muscles. When muscles become tight, what actually happens is that lactic acid gets accumulated in them.

Under ordinary conditions, when a muscle works, glucose gets converted into carbon dioxide and water. The blood easily removes these two waste materials.

But when a muscle has to work for too long, the energy demand is too high that the cells do not get time to convert glucose fully into carbon dioxide and water. Instead, the glucose is converted into another substance that is lactic acid.

The problem with lactic acid is that it restricts further movement of the muscles and results in muscular cramps. In such conditions, application of a little bit of pressure can help the muscles release the pent up lactic acid. When the cervical and neck muscles get accumulated with lactic acid, it often results in a headache. The exercise that is described below can prove to be very effective.

1. Turn on the shower and direct the flow of the stream of warm water onto the back of your neck.

2. Now turn your head as if you are trying to see who is behind you.

3. Stand like this for one or two minute.

4. Then repeat the exercise but looking in the opposite side this time.

Tip 96.

Take naps. A 20 minute power nap during your lunch break will give your body the extra boost it needs to continue throughout the day with less tension. It will also allow you to be refreshed and without as many worries.

Tip 97.

Eat organic foods. Many foods especially produce and meat, contain pesticides and hormones that are not good for the body. More and more stores are carrying organic foods that are safer for your body and reduce the number of foreign chemicals entering into your bloodstream. If your local grocery store does not carry any of these food items, check to see if your city has an organic store somewhere else.

Tip 98.

See a massage therapist. Massage therapist are experts in knowing how to work out tight muscles in the body. They know which muscles of the neck are the major contributors to tension headaches and know excellent techniques for stretching those specific muscles. Having massages regularly is a great way to relieve muscle tension and prevent headaches.

Tip 99.

See a chiropractor. You knew it was coming. I had to throw in good word for my profession. Chiropractic care is a safe, effective treatment for *all* types of headaches. Chiropractors can examine your spine and musculature, including that of the neck, to determine if there are any issues that could possibly be causing headaches to occur. They can perform a spinal adjustment that will provide relief and help prevent the onset of future headaches.

Congratulations! You have read through all 99 Natural Ways to Beat a Headache! Now you should be able to understand some of the possible

www.ingramcontent.com/pod-product-compliance
Lightning Source LLC
LaVergne TN
LVHW041300150826
845673LV00008B/2666

* 9 7 9 8 7 3 2 0 0 8 0 4 3 *